TABLE OF CONTENTS

The Face of Anorexia
Approximately 95% of Those Affected by Anorexia Are Females – Learn Why?
©Copyright 2013 By Dr. Harry Jay

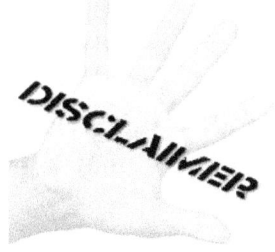

DISCLAIMER AND TERMS OF USE AGREEMENT:

(Please Read This Before Using This Book)

This information is for educational and informational purposes only. The content is not intended to be a substitute for any professional advice, diagnosis, or treatment.

The authors and publisher of this book and the accompanying materials have used their best efforts in preparing this book.

The authors and publisher make no representation or warranties with respect to the accuracy, applicability, fitness, or completeness of the contents of this book. The information contained in this book is strictly for educational purposes. Therefore, if you wish to apply ideas contained in this book, you are taking full responsibility for your actions.

Introduction

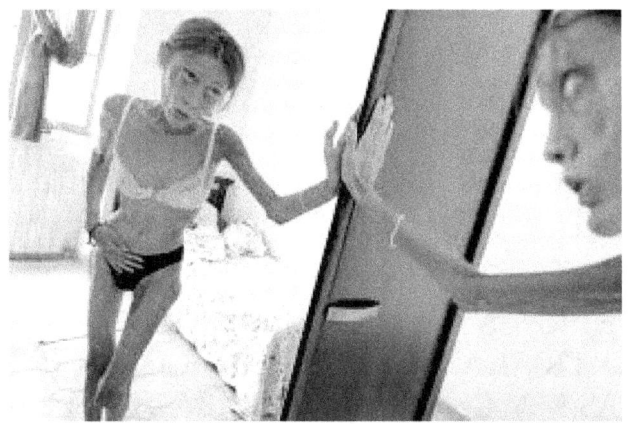

This is not an easy subject to understand and discuss. It is painful to understand and witness this disease as it affects your loved ones and friends.

All diseases and disorders are horrific and anorexia or as the medical community calls it "Anorexia Nervosa" is no exception. The cover photo is enough to make you pause and hold back a few emotions.

My name is Dr. Harry Jay and I've been a behavioral scientist for over 32-years. Of the hundreds of anorexia patients I have counseled, none of them have been easy. The problem is not going to go away without some serious consideration as to how the problem begins. I will be discussing all aspects of anorexia throughout this book.

Statistics show that anorexia confronts both males and females but over 95% of all anorexia patients are teenage girls. Today, teenage peer pressure is at an all time high. As I write this introduction, the evening news is reporting that teenage girls are now going online and asking strangers to critique their looks. If this isn't a massive cultivation of anorexia seeds then I don't know what is!

Being concerned with one's looks is not new and vanity has been with us from the dawn of mankind. What is new is the type of society that we now live in that is dedicated to good looks, beauty, bodybuilding, and fitness and exercise to a point where it becomes problematic.

THERE IS NOTHING WRONG WITH BEING FIT AND TRIM AND LOOKING GOOD UNLESS IT BECOMES AN OBSESSION AND BECOMES PROBLEMATIC!

In today's society of consumerism and entertainment, we constantly want more and we constantly want to be entertained and we constantly want it NOW! Gain of any type comes by sacrifice but today's young people are growing up in single parent homes and if they are lucky enough to have two parents then both are working long hours just to get by with the last thing on their mind being problems with their kids.

In a recent interview with what seemed a perfectly normal family, the mother broke down in tears anguishing over the fact that she doesn't have time for the things that are important to her. Where have I heard this before?

Parents – you need to stay active with your kids; know their friends, know who they associate with, where they hang out, and keep in close contact with their school administrators and teachers.

Teenagers need boundaries and these boundaries are such that only parents can provide them. Adolescence is tough and these are the most formidable years.

Decisions made during adolescence, habits formed and beliefs acquired stay with an individual for a lifetime if not corrected.

Maturity plays a big factor here and especially with teenage girls who are highly susceptible to criticism and bullying by other teenage girls.

So, let's begin with one important fact about anorexia…

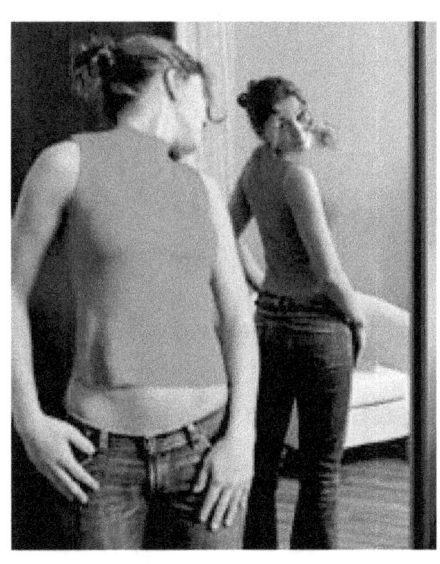

Anorexia doesn't just HAPPEN!

The telltale signs can be observed way in advance before it becomes a severe mental problem. I will outline the signs for you so that you will be armed and ready to spot this horrific problem before it becomes acute.

So to begin, allow me to define what anorexia nervosa is: anorexia nervosa is a type of eating disorder and people who have anorexia have an <u>intense fear</u> of gaining weight. They severely limit the amount of food they eat and often engage in severe workout programs that may encompass up to four hours per day.

Anorexia is NOT a physical disease; anorexia is a mental disorder that affects the physical body.

Anorexia nervosa has the highest death rate of any mental illness. Between 5% and 20% of people who develop the disease will eventually die from it.

Anorexia is not about weight or food!

Believe it or not, anorexia isn't really about weight and food - at least not at its core. Eating disorders are much more complicated than that.

The food and weight-related issues are symptoms of something deeper: things like depression, loneliness, insecurity, pressure to be perfect, or feeling out of control.

Things that no amount of dieting or weight loss can cure; in other words, anorexia is the EFFECT of some underlying problem!

Types of anorexia nervosa

There are two types of anorexia.

1. In the **restricting type** of anorexia, weight loss is achieved by restricting calories (following drastic diets, fasting, and exercising to excess).

2. In the **purging type** of anorexia, weight loss is achieved by vomiting or using laxatives and diuretics. Bulimia is the result!

Are you anorexic?

- Do you feel fat even though people tell you you're not?

- Are you terrified of gaining weight?

- Do you lie about how much you eat or hide your eating habits from others?

- Are your friends or family concerned about your weight loss, eating habits, or appearance?

- Do you diet, compulsively exercise, or purge when you're feeling overwhelmed or bad about yourself?

- Do you feel powerful or in control when you go without food, over-exercise, or purge?

- Do you base your self-worth on your weight or body size?

What causes anorexia?

Eating disorders are complex, and behavioral scientists don't really know what causes them. But they may be due to a mix of family history, social factors, and personality traits. You may be more likely to have anorexia if:

- Other people in your family have an eating disorder, such as anorexia or bulimia nervosa.

- You have a job or do a sport that stresses body size, such as ballet, modeling, or gymnastics.

- You are the type of person who tries to be perfect all the time, never feels good enough, or worries a lot.

- You are dealing with stressful life events, such as divorce, moving to a new town or school, or losing a loved one.

What are the symptoms?

People who have anorexia are often strongly in denial that they have a problem. They don't see or believe that they do. It's usually up to their loved ones to get help for them. If you are worried about someone, you can look for certain signs.

People who have anorexia:

- Weigh much less than is healthy or normal.

- Are very afraid of gaining weight.

- Refuse to stay at a normal weight.

- Think they are overweight even when they are very thin.

Their lives become focused on controlling their weight. They may:

- Obsess about food, weight, and dieting.
- Strictly limit how much they eat.
- Exercise a lot, even when they are sick.
- Vomit or use laxatives or water pills (diuretics) to avoid weight gain.

Common feelings and actions that are linked to anorexia nervosa include.

- Having an intense fear of gaining weight.
- Restricting food or types of food, such as food that contains any kind of fat or sugar.
- Weighing less than 85% of your expected body weight. (In a child or teen, losing or not gaining weight during a growth spurt is not good.)
- Seeing your body as overweight, in spite of being underweight or a distorted body image.
- Exercising too much.
- Being secretive around food and not recognizing or wanting to talk about having a problem with eating or weight loss.

Some people who have anorexia also make themselves vomit or use laxatives or diuretics to lose weight (bulimia). Breakdown of the enamel on the teeth is a common symptom of long-term vomiting/purging.

Physical signs

Common physical signs of malnutrition from anorexia include:

- A low body weight.

- Constipation and slow emptying of the stomach.

- Thinning hair, dry skin, and brittle nails.

- Shrunken breasts.

- Stopping or never getting a monthly menstrual period.

- Feeling cold, with a lower-than-normal body temperature.

- Low blood pressure.

Food rituals

People who have anorexia often form rituals associated with eating. These may include:

- Developing special ways to eat food, hoarding food, collecting recipes, and preparing elaborate meals for other people but not eating the meals themselves.

- Spending a lot of time cutting and rearranging food on their plates to make it look as though they have eaten. They may also hide food or secretly get rid of it during meals.

Suicidal feelings

In some cases, people who have eating disorders can feel suicidal.

- Warning signs of possible suicide in children and teens can include making suicide threats, being preoccupied with death or suicide, giving away belongings, withdrawing, being angry, or having failing grades.

- Warning signs and possible triggers of suicide in adults can include making suicide threats, alcohol or substance abuse, depression, giving away belongings, a recent job loss, or divorce.

How is anorexia diagnosed?

If your doctor thinks that you may have an eating disorder, he or she will compare your weight with the expected weight for someone of your height and age. He or she will also check your heart, lungs, blood pressure, skin, and hair to look for problems caused by not eating enough. You may also have blood tests or X-rays.

Your doctor may ask questions about how you feel. It is common for a treatable mental health problem such as depression or anxiety to play a part in an eating disorder.

How is it treated?

All people who have anorexia need treatment. Even if you or someone you care about has only a couple of the signs of an eating disorder, get help now. Early treatment gives the best chance of overcoming anorexia.

13

Treatment can help you get back to and stay at a healthy weight. It can also help you learn good eating habits and learn to feel better about yourself. Because anorexia is both a physical and emotional problem, you may work with a doctor, a dietitian, and a counselor.

If your weight has dropped too low, you will need to be treated in a hospital.

Anorexia can take a long time to overcome, and it is common to fall back into unhealthy habits. If you are having problems, don't try to handle them on your own. Get help now.

What should you do if you think someone has anorexia?

It can be very scary to realize that someone you care about has an eating disorder. But you can help.

If you think your child has anorexia:

- Talk to her. Tell her why you are worried. Let her know you care.

- Make an appointment for you and your child to meet with a doctor or a counselor.

If you're worried about someone you know:

- Tell someone who can make a difference, like a parent, teacher, counselor, or doctor. A person with anorexia may insist that she doesn't need help, but she does. The sooner she gets treatment, the sooner she will be healthy again.

14

Being diagnosed

There is no single test that can diagnose anorexia. But this illness has a visible effect on your health and eating habits.

If your doctor thinks that you may have an eating disorder, he or she will check you for signs of malnutrition or starvation. Your doctor may also ask questions about your mental well-being. It is common for a treatable mental health problem (such as depression, anxiety, or obsessive-compulsive disorder) to play a part in an eating disorder.

Exams and Tests

Common exams and tests for a possible eating disorder include:

- A medical history of your physical and emotional health, present and past.

- A physical exam, including checking your heart, lungs, blood pressure, weight, mouth, skin, and hair for problems from malnutrition.

- Screening questions about your eating habits and how you feel about your health.

- A mental health assessment, to check for depression or anxiety.

- Blood tests, to check for signs of malnutrition.

- X-rays, which can show whether your bones have been weakened (osteopenia) by malnutrition.

If your doctor thinks that you may have organ damage, doing heart or kidney tests can be helpful.

Other causes of weight loss or muscle wasting must be ruled out with medical testing. Examples of other conditions that can cause these symptoms include:

- Addison's disease
- Celiac disease
- Inflammatory bowel disease

Tests should be done to help find the cause of weight loss, or see what damage the weight loss has caused. Many of these tests will be repeated over time to monitor the patient.

These tests may include:

- Albumin
- Bone density test to check for thin bones (osteoporosis)
- CBC
- Electrocardiogram (ECG or EKG)
- Electrolytes
- Kidney function tests
- Liver function tests
- Total protein
- Thyroid function tests
- Urinalysis

Getting treatment

All people with anorexia need treatment. In most cases, this involves seeing a doctor and having regular counseling sessions. A hospital stay is needed for those who are seriously underweight or who have severe medical problems. The goals of treatment are to restore a healthy weight and healthy eating habits.

If you have an eating disorder, try not to resist treatment. Although you may be very afraid of gaining weight, try to think of weight gain as a life-saving measure. With help, you can learn to eat well and keep your weight at a healthy level.

The biggest challenge in treating anorexia nervosa is making the person recognize that they have an illness. Most persons with anorexia nervosa deny that they have an eating disorder. People often enter treatment only once their condition is serious.

The goals of treatment are to restore normal body weight and eating habits. A weight gain of 1 - 3 pounds per week is considered a safe goal.

A number of different programs have been designed to treat anorexia. Sometimes the person can gain weight by:

- Increasing social activity
- Reducing physical activity
- Using schedules for eating

Many patients start with a short hospital stay and continue to follow-up with a day treatment program.

A longer hospital stay may be needed if:

- The person has lost a lot of weight (being below 70% of their ideal body weight for their age and height). For severe and life-threatening malnutrition, the person may need to be fed through a vein or stomach tube.

- Weight loss continues even with treatment
- Medical complications, such as heart problems, confusion, or low potassium levels develop
- The person has severe depression or thinks about committing suicide

Care providers who are usually involved in these programs include:

- Nurse practitioners
- Physicians
- Nutritionists or dietitians
- Mental health care providers

Treatment is often very difficult, and patients and their families must work hard. Many therapies may be tried until the patient overcomes this disorder.

Patients may drop out of programs if they have unrealistic hopes of being "cured" with therapy alone.

Different kinds of talk therapy are used to treat people with anorexia:

- Individual cognitive behavioral therapy, group therapy, and family therapy have all been successful.
- The goal of therapy is to change a patient's thoughts or behavior to encourage them to eat in a healthier way. This kind of therapy is

more useful for treating younger patients who have not had anorexia for a long time.

- If the patient is young, therapy may involve the whole family. The family is seen as a part of the solution, instead of the cause of the eating disorder.

- Support groups may also be a part of treatment. In support groups, patients and families meet and share what they've been through.

Medications such as antidepressants, antipsychotics, and mood stabilizers may help some anorexic patients when given as part of a complete treatment program. Examples include:

- Antidepressants

- Olanzapine (Zyprexa, Zydis)

- Selective serotonin reuptake inhibitors (SSRIs)

These medicines can help treat depression or anxiety.

Although these drugs may help, no medication has been proven to decrease the desire to lose weight.

Possible Complications

Complications can be severe. A hospital stay may be needed.

Complications may include:

- Bloating or swelling

- Bone weakening

- Electrolyte imbalance (such as low potassium)
- Dangerous heart rhythms
- Decrease in white blood cells, which leads to increased risk of infection
- Severe dehydration
- Severe malnutrition
- Seizures due to fluid loss from repeated diarrhea or vomiting
- Thyroid gland problems, which can lead to cold intolerance and constipation
- Tooth decay

Your recovery

Ideally, you can take charge of anorexia with the help of a team that includes a mental health professional (such as a psychologist or licensed counselor), a medical health professional (such as a doctor or nurse), and a registered dietitian.

If your medical condition is not life-threatening, your treatment likely will include:

- **Medical treatment.** If malnutrition or starvation has started to break down your body, medical treatment will be a top priority. Your doctor will treat the medical conditions that have been caused by anorexia, such as osteoporosis, heart problems, or depression. As you begin to get better, your doctor will continue to follow your health and weight.

- **Nutritional counseling.** A registered dietitian will help you take charge of your weight in a healthy way. You will learn healthy eating patterns and gain a good understanding of nutrition.

An important part of your recovery will include:

- **Taking control of your eating habits**.

- **Learning emotional self-care**.

- **Building trust in people who are trying to help you**.

For the teen with anorexia, family involvement is a key part of treatment. Family therapy helps parents support their child, both emotionally and physically. It also supports parents in creating a normal eating pattern for their child. Any brothers or sisters also need support during treatment. Family, group, and individual counseling are all effective and are often combined.

If you need more help

Ongoing (chronic) forms of anorexia may require treatment for many years, including hospitalizations when needed. Ongoing treatment usually includes psychological counseling. A counselor will help you make your own plan to use new coping and stress management skills and prevent relapse. Your counselor can help you at those times when it is hard to follow healthy ways of thinking about food and your body.

Some people fully recover from anorexia. Many people with anorexia have ups and downs over the years. Try thinking of treatment as an ongoing process.

When you need emergency care

Being severely underweight can cause dehydration, starvation, and electrolyte imbalance, any of which can be life-threatening.

If anorexia causes life-threatening medical problems, you need urgent medical treatment. Treatment in a hospital or eating disorder treatment center will first include:

- **Treating starvation.** This can include treating medical problems it has caused, such as dehydration, electrolyte imbalance, or heart problems. If you can't eat, you are given your nutrition in fluid form.

- **Nutritional rehabilitation.** The medical team helps you work toward a healthier weight carefully and gradually, learn when your body is hungry and full, and start healthy eating patterns.

If you are 15% below your healthy weight or thinner, you will benefit from a structured treatment program to help you get better. In some cases, a treatment program can take 2 to 6 months.

You may need hospitalization if you weigh 25% below your healthy weight. For example, if your lowest healthy weight is 125 lb (57 kg) and you drop to about 100 lb (45 kg), you will need inpatient treatment. This can include several weeks in the hospital followed by outpatient treatment to monitor your progress.

What to Think About

Anorexia can be a lifelong illness. Many people who have anorexia recover, some improve, and some have problems with anorexia throughout their lives.

- People with anorexia who are young and who start treatment early in their illness usually do well.

- Anorexia is more difficult to treat when it has gone untreated for a long time.

Many people don't get treatment for mental health problems. You may not seek treatment because you think your symptoms are not bad enough or that you can work things out on your own. But getting treatment is important.

If you need help deciding whether to see your doctor, read about some reasons why people don't get help and how to overcome them.

Who is at risk for anorexia nervosa?

Approximately 95% of those affected by anorexia are female, most often teenage girls, but males can develop the disorder as well. While anorexia typically begins to manifest itself during early adolescence, it is also seen in young children and adults. In the U.S. and other countries with high economic status, it is estimated that about one out of every 100 adolescent girls has the disorder. Caucasians are more often affected than people of other racial backgrounds, and anorexia is more common in middle and upper socioeconomic groups. According to the U.S. National Institute of Mental Health (NIMH), other statistics about this disorder include the fact that an estimated 0.5%-3.7% of women will suffer from this disorder at some point in their lives. About 0.3% of men are thought to develop anorexia in their lifetimes

Many experts consider people for whom thinness is especially desirable, or a professional requirement (such as athletes, models, dancers, and actors), to be at risk for eating disorders such as anorexia nervosa. Health-care professionals are usually encouraged to present the facts about the dangers of anorexia through education of their patients and of the general public as a means of preventing this and other eating disorders.

What causes anorexia nervosa?

At this time, no definite cause of anorexia nervosa has been determined. However, research within the medical and psychological fields continues to explore possible causes.

Studies suggest that a genetic (inherited) component may play a more significant role in determining a person's susceptibility to anorexia than was previously thought. Researchers are currently attempting to identify the particular gene or genes that might affect a person's tendency to develop this disorder, and preliminary studies suggest that a gene located at chromosome 1p seems to be involved in determining a person's susceptibility to anorexia nervosa.

Other evidence had pinpointed a dysfunction in the part of the brain, the hypothalamus (which regulates certain metabolic processes), as contributing to the development of anorexia. Other studies have suggested that imbalances in neurotransmitter (brain chemicals involved in signaling and regulatory processes) levels in the brain may occur in people suffering from anorexia.

Feeding problems as an infant, a general history of under eating and maternal depressive symptoms tend to be risk factors for developing anorexia. Other personal characteristics that can predispose an individual to the development of anorexia include a high level of negative feelings and perfectionism. For many individuals with anorexia, the destructive cycle begins with the pressure to be thin and attractive. A poor self-image compounds the problem. People who suffer from any eating disorder are more likely to have been the victim of childhood abuse.

While some professionals remain of the opinion that family discord and high demands from parents can put a person at risk for developing this disorder, the increasing evidence against the idea that families cause anorexia has mounted to such an extent that professional mental-health organizations no longer ascribe to that theory. Possible factors that protect against the development of anorexia include high maternal body mass index (BMI) as well as personal high self-esteem.

The exact causes of anorexia nervosa are unknown. Many factors probably are involved. Genes and hormones may play a role. Social attitudes promoting very thin body types may also be involved.

Family conflicts are no longer thought to contribute to this or other eating disorders.

Risk factors for anorexia include:

- Trying to be perfect or overly focused on rules
- Being more worried about, or paying more attention to, weight and shape
- Having eating problems during infancy or early childhood
- Certain social or cultural ideas about health and beauty
- Having a negative self-image
- Having an anxiety disorder as a child

Anorexia usually begins during the teen years or young adulthood. It is more common in females, but may also be seen in males. The disorder is seen mainly in white women who are high academic achievers and who have a goal-oriented family or personality.

When to Contact a Medical Professional

Talk to your doctor if a loved one is:

- Too focused on weight
- Over-exercising
- Limiting his or her food intake
- Very underweight

Getting medical help right away can make an eating disorder less severe.

Prevention

In some cases, prevention may not be possible. Encouraging healthy, realistic attitudes toward weight and diet may be helpful. Sometimes, talk therapy can help.

The Psychology of Anorexia

People with anorexia are often perfectionists and overachievers. They're the "good" daughters and sons who do what they're told, excel in everything they do, and focus on pleasing others. But while they may appear to have it all together, inside they feel helpless, inadequate, and worthless. Through their harshly critical lens, if they're not perfect, they're a total failure.

Family and social pressures

In addition to the cultural pressure to be thin, there are other family and social pressures that can contribute to anorexia. This includes participation in an activity that demands slenderness, such as ballet, gymnastics, or modeling. It also includes having parents who are overly controlling, put a lot of emphasis on looks, diet themselves, or criticize their children's bodies and appearance. Stressful life events—such as the onset of puberty, a breakup, or going away to school—can also trigger anorexia.

Biological causes of anorexia

Research suggests that a genetic predisposition to anorexia may run in families. If a girl has a sibling with anorexia, she is 10 to 20 times more likely than the general population to develop

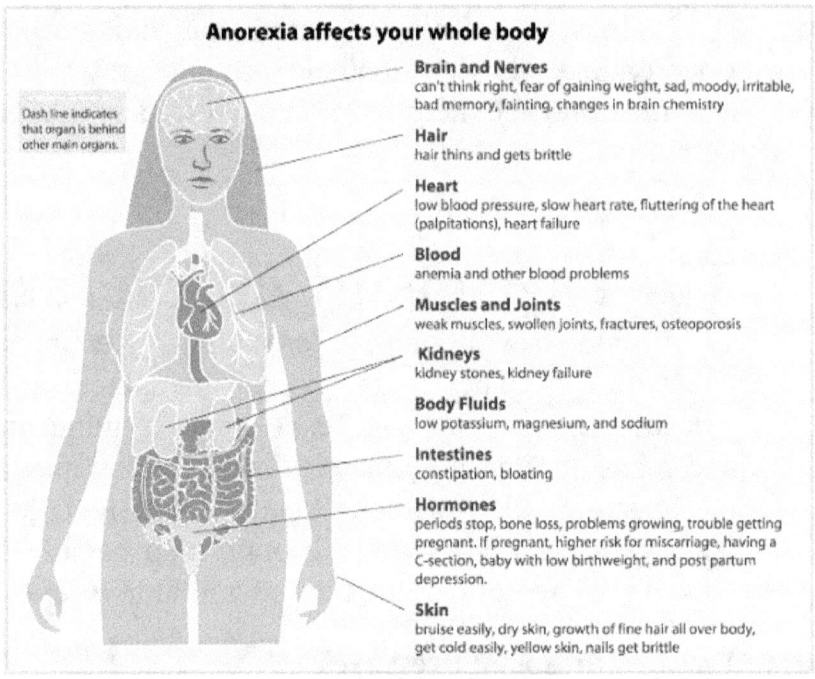

Anorexia affects your whole body

Dash line indicates that organ is behind other main organs.

Brain and Nerves
can't think right, fear of gaining weight, sad, moody, irritable, bad memory, fainting, changes in brain chemistry

Hair
hair thins and gets brittle

Heart
low blood pressure, slow heart rate, fluttering of the heart (palpitations), heart failure

Blood
anemia and other blood problems

Muscles and Joints
weak muscles, swollen joints, fractures, osteoporosis

Kidneys
kidney stones, kidney failure

Body Fluids
low potassium, magnesium, and sodium

Intestines
constipation, bloating

Hormones
periods stop, bone loss, problems growing, trouble getting pregnant. If pregnant, higher risk for miscarriage, having a C-section, baby with low birthweight, and post partum depression.

Skin
bruise easily, dry skin, growth of fine hair all over body, get cold easily, yellow skin, nails get brittle

Energy Psychology may correct the problem

The following treatment protocol has had some amazing success in treating all types of eating disorders and can be administered by anyone other than the anorexic. It employs the body's own energy to realign the mind's belief systems. It is simple and safe and is not hocus pocus!

Eating disorders—a group of mental disorders including anorexia nervosa, bulimia nervosa, pica, and a rumination disorder in infancy

As a group of disorders, it is characterized by physiological and psychological disturbances in appetite and food consumption. It seems that almost always, the sufferer may not be aware mentally that they have a problem. Characterized by self-induced weight loss, negative perception of body-image, self-induced vomiting, strict dieting or fasting, vigorous exercise, or use of laxatives or diuretics, these problems may disrupt homeostasis for the entire body, causing lasting destruction.

Eating Disorders interfere with living an abundant life.

Why does she think I'm skinny? I've never looked bigger.

She goes to the bathroom after every slice of pizza. What is going on with her?

I haven't had my period in months, and now my hair is falling out in clumps.

If I could just lose ten more pounds, I would be so happy.

Maybe I can get my doctor to prescribe the water pill for me. This excess weight has to be water!

Are these problems? Absolutely! Are these *the* problem? *NEVER!*

Energy Psychology changes the heart pictures behind the Eating Disorders.

Informed Consent

These techniques are not intended to diagnose, prescribe, treat, or cure any disease whether physical or mental. These techniques are self-help techniques used for balancing bio-energetic systems, relaxation, and stress reduction and are not intended as a substitute for regular medical care. No action or inaction should be taken based solely on the contents herein; instead, readers or viewers should consult appropriate health professionals on any matter relating to their health. This information has not been evaluated by the FDA and we make no curative claims. We only relate the reported experience of clients and pre- and post-Heart Rate Variability tests. This information and the opinion provided here are believed to be accurate and sound, based on the best judgment, experience, and research of the author. Readers or viewers who fail to consult with appropriate health authorities assume the risk of any injuries. Using the techniques herein is acknowledging that you have read, understand, and agree to this disclaimer and therefore that informed consent has been established. DO NOT USE THE TECHNIQUES IF YOU DO NOT AGREE TO THE LAST SENTENCE.

Getting Started

☐ Read, understand and agree to the Informed Consent Section of the disclaimer on this card. By doing the self-treatment, you are agreeing to the Informed Consent clause.

☐ Thoroughly read the materials provided

☐ Have something to write with and write on.

☐ Find a quiet setting where you can relax and focus on healing.

☐ Familiarize yourself with the instructions below for completing the Resonating Memory Pictures.

☐ Complete the Resonating Memory Pictures.

Resonating Memory Pictures Worksheet

The issue I'm working on:

_____

*Visualizing and identifying thoughts and feelings can, and will in some cases, speed up the process of healing. This is why we encourage you to do so if you are able, but it is not a requirement for success. All of our validating data was gathered from individuals who did NOT use any visualization techniques during their protocol sessions. **If you have trouble visualizing your pictures during a protocol session, saying or describing these pictures can work just as well.***

1. Identify a Current Picture of how this issue currently manifests itself. (*for example*, the issue I'm working on is anger. The current picture is being short-tempered with my family at the dinner table since losing my job last month).

Rate the intensity from 0-10 (with 0 being the least intense and 10 being the most intense) of the emotion you feel when you think about the issue you are working on.

What thoughts and emotions do you have when focusing on your Current Picture? (*for example*, hopeless, angry, confused)

How do you think and feel about others and the world when focusing on your Current Picture? (*for example*, I don't have a place in this world, no one understands me, it's a cruel world, people only care about themselves)

2. **Identify an Early Picture** of when you can recall experiencing similar thoughts and feelings as those listed for your current picture. (*This should be the earliest time you remember experiencing similar thoughts and feelings, not the first time you experienced the same situation. For example*, my parent's divorce).

Rate the intensity from 0-10 (with 0 being the least intense and 10 being the most intense) of the emotion you feel when you think about your earliest picture.

What thoughts and emotions do you have when focusing on your Earliest Picture? (*for example*, hopeless, angry, confused)

How do you think and feel about others and the world when focusing on your Earliest Picture? (*for example*, I don't have a place in this world, no one understands me, it's a cruel world, people only care about themselves)

3. Identify a Love Picture by thinking of one or more individuals in your life from whom you felt deep love. These can be people from the past or present. (friends, family, etc.) You may also include God on this list.

Picture yourself surrounded and loved by those on your "love list." Picture them one at a time, or as a whole group. Relax and enjoy feeling their love touch your heart.

EATING DISORDERS PROTOCOLS

INSTRUCTIONS: Throughout each protocol session, focus alternately on the **Early Picture** you found while completing the Resonating Memory Pictures and your **Love Picture**. If you indentified more than one **Early Picture**, use the earliest one. If you are unable to find an **Early Picture**, focus on healing your **Current Picture**. If you are unable to find a **Love Picture**, imagine yourself surrounded by people you love and people who love you including God, if that fits your belief system. Once your **Early Picture** reaches an intensity of zero (0), complete the Resonating Memory Pictures process again to find your next earliest picture.

Follow each of these steps:

☐ Complete the following **Eating Disorders Protocol** for the specified number of minutes and specified times per day.

- ☐ Complete the **Booster Protocol** (*after completing the Eating Disorders Protocol*) for the specified number of minutes and specified times per day.

- ☐ Continue the **Eating Disorders Protocol** and **Booster Protocol** for as long as necessary until the intensity of either the **Early Picture** or **Current Picture** you are focusing on reaches zero (0).

- ☐ Consider your Eating Disorders issue. If it is resolved, move to using just the **Eating Disorders Protocol Maintenance** every day.

  If it is unresolved, complete the Resonating Memory Pictures again to find another **Early Picture** on which to focus. Then continue doing the **Eating Disorders Protocol** and **Booster Protocol** for that new picture. Repeat this entire process as many times as necessary until the Eating Disorders issue is resolved.

Eating Disorders Protocol

On the bridge of your nose, place the palm-side, 2nd section of your RH thumb. On the left side of your neck, place all of your LH prints. 2 minute! 2 times/week! *5 times/week maximum*

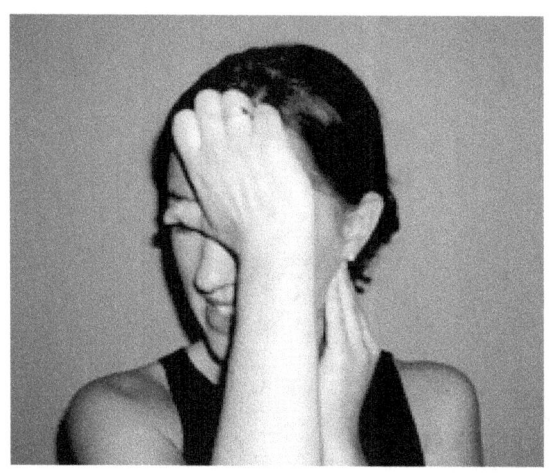

<u>Eating Disorders Protocol Maintenance</u>

Once your issue is resolved, it is important to continue using these protocols daily for maintenance. Daily work is critical to keep the autonomic nervous system in balance, and to prevent the return of your issue. Either continue daily work using the following maintenance protocol, or choose another Theolegions treatment to use. You may discontinue the maintenance protocol if you begin using another Theolegions treatment. To maximize the benefit of this work in your life, it is recommended that you choose another issue to work on.

On the bridge of your nose, place the palm-side, 2nd section of your RH thumb. On the left side of your neck, place all of your LH prints. 1 minute. 2 times/week. *5 times/week maximum*

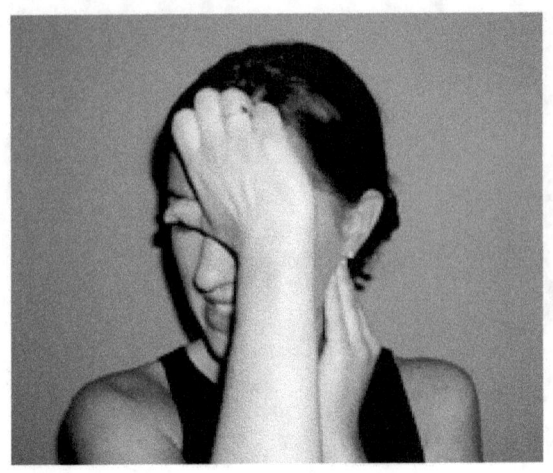

BOOSTER PROTOCOL

On the front of your neck, place your whole LH. On the back of your neck, place your RH. Thumb print. Middle finger nail. Ring finger nail. 3 minutes

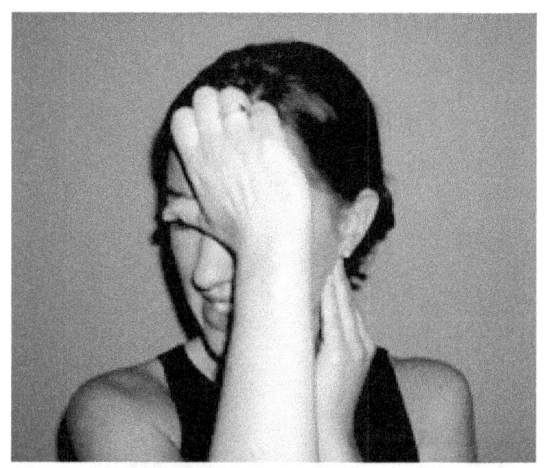

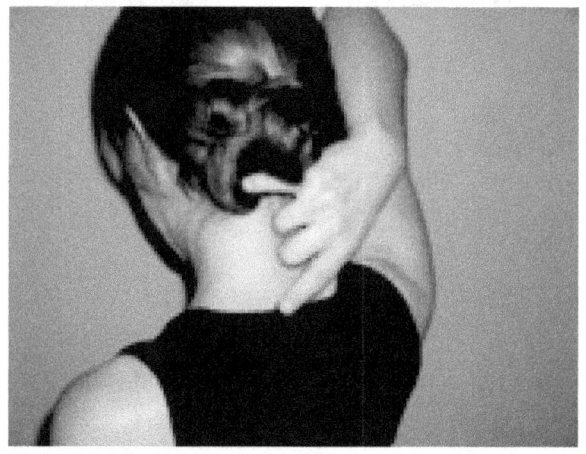

On the back of your neck, place all of your RH nails. On the front of your neck, place your LH. Thumb nail. Middle finger nail. Little finger nail. 2 minutes. 2 times/day. *(4 times/day maximum)*

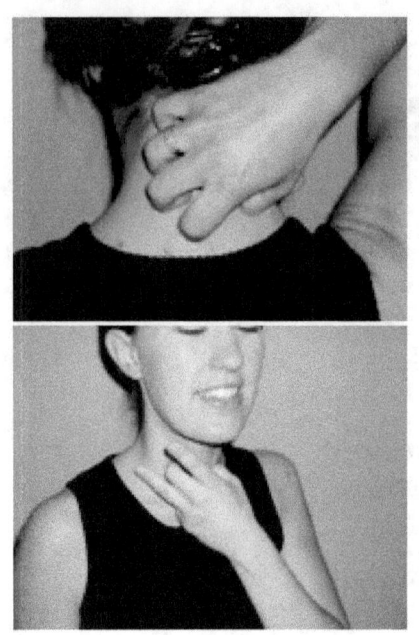

I Have a Special Gift for My Readers

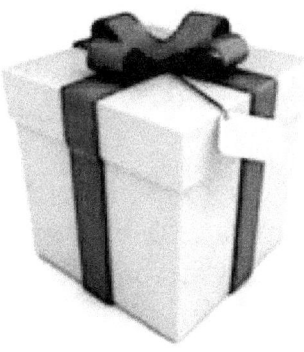

I appreciate my readers for without them I am just another author attempting to make a difference. If my book has made a favorable impression please leave me an honest review. Thank you in advance for you participation.

My readers and I have in common a passion for the written word as well as the desire to learn and grow from books.

My special offer to you is a massive ebook library that I have compiled over the years. It contains hundreds of fiction and non-fiction ebooks in Adobe Acrobat PDF format as well as the Greek classics and old literary classics too.

In fact, this library is so massive to completely download the entire library will require over 5 GBs open on your desktop.

Use the link below and scan all of the ebooks in the library. You can select the ebooks you want individually or download the entire library.

The link below does not expire after a given time period so you are free to return for more books rather than clog your desktop. And feel free to give the link to your friends who enjoy reading too.

I thank you for reading my book and hope if you are pleased that you will leave me an honest review so that I can improve my work and or write books that appeal to your interests.

Okay, here is the link…

http://tinyurl.com/special-readers-promo

PS: If you wish to reach me personally for any reason you may simply write to mailto:support@epubwealth.com.

I answer all of my emails so rest assured I will respond.

Meet the Author

Dr. Harry Jay is Director of Research for AppliedMindSciences.com, a mental health and mind research group of Applied Web Info, and is the author of over 100 books and research papers as a behavioral scientist.

In his 32-year career, Dr. Harry Jay has contributed many new mental health treatment treatments and protocols using some of the new advances he has discovered in Energy Psychology.

He specializes in addictions of all kinds, sexual abuse, child predation and gender relationships.

He is also a board member to ePubWealth.com and serves on the science committee assisting non-fiction science writers in book publishing and promotion.

As a leading behavioral scientist, he provides profiling services to the company's ForensicsNation.com unit as well as criminal psychology research to aid in identifying and apprehending child predators and cyber-criminals of all kinds.

He resides in Southern Utah and enjoys the outdoors, fishing and photography.

Visit some of his websites
http://www.AddMeInNow.com
http://www.AppliedMindSciences.com
http://www.AppliedWebInfo.com
http://www.BookbuilderPLUS.com
http://www.BookJumping.com
http://www.EmailNations.com
http://www.EmbarrassingProblemsFix.com
http://www.ePubWealth.com
http://www.ForensicsNation.com
http://www.ForensicsNationStore.com
http://www.FreebiesNation.com
http://www.HealthFitnessWellnessNation.com
http://www.Neternatives.com
http://www.PrivacyNations.com
http://www.RetireWithoutMoney.org
http://www.SurvivalNations.com
http://www.TheBentonKitchen.com
http://www.Theolegions.org
http://www.VideoBookbuilder.com

Some Other Books You May Enjoy From ePubWealth.com, LLC Library Catalog

EPW Library Catalog Online
http://www.epubwealth.com/wp-content/uploads/2013/07/Leland-benton-private-turbo.pdf

EPW Library Catalog Download
http://www.filefactory.com/f/562ef3ea1a054f0a

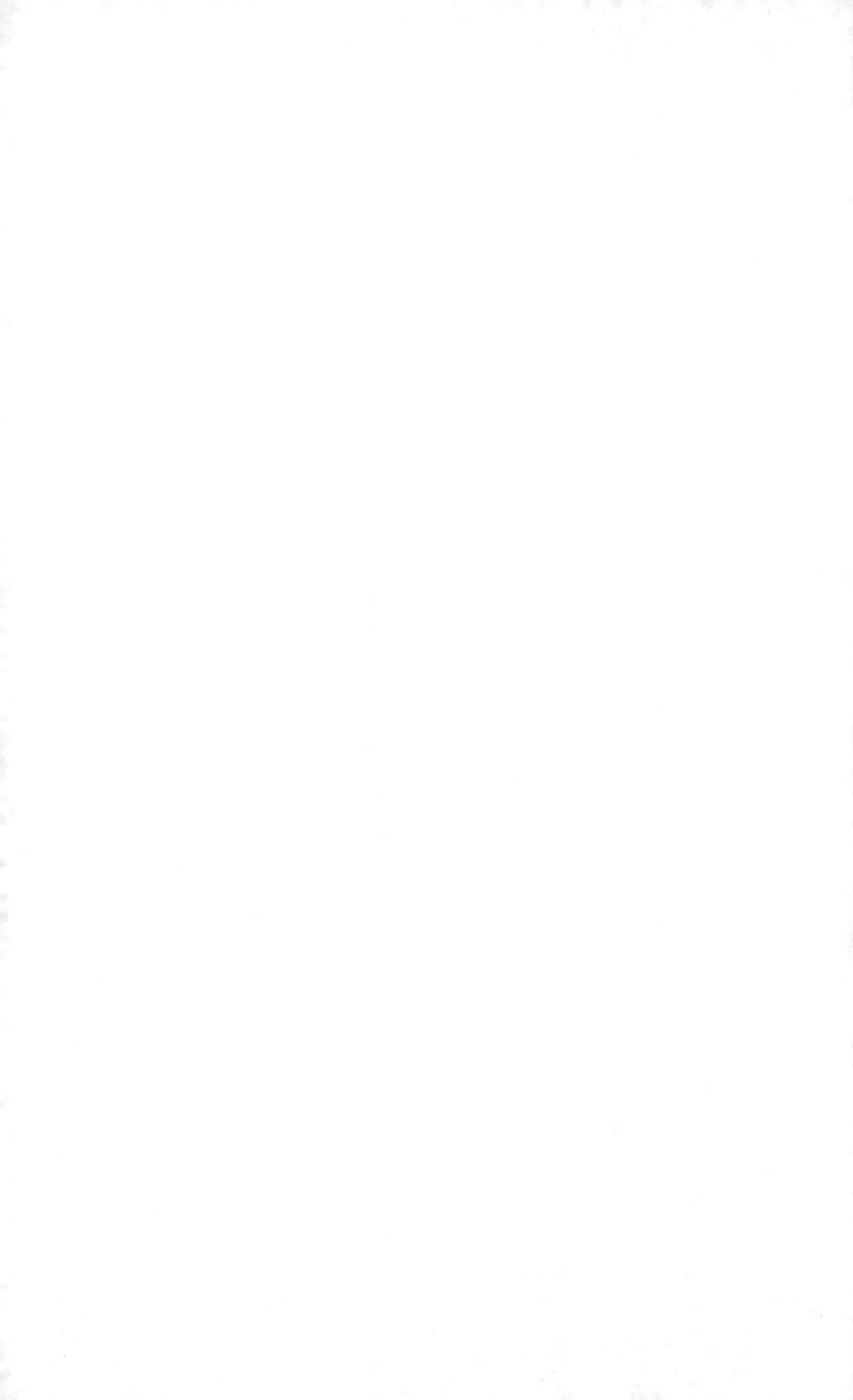